CONTENTS

1. 01. No-bake keto desserts: Peanut butter chocolate bars   1
2. 02. Keto cake – (The best chocolate recipe)   4
3. 03. Low carb keto cream cheese cookies   6
4. 04. Keto lemon bars   8
5. 05. 3 Ingredient Keto Chocolate Coconut Cups   10
6. 06. Peanut Butter Mousse – Keto and Sugar-Free   14
7. 07. Keto No-Bake Cookies   16
8. 08. Keto Chocolate Chip Cookies   18
9. 09. Keto Cheesecake Brownies   21
10. 10. Best Ever Keto Chocolate Cake   24
11. 11. Nut-Free Keto Brownie   26
12. 12. Easy Keto Chocolate Frosty   28
13. 13. Easy Keto Muffins   30
14. 14. No-Bake Keto Chocolate Chip Cookie Bars   32
15. 15. Low Carb Lemon Mousse Recipe   35
16. 16. Keto Chocolate Cheesecake Bites   37
17. 17. Keto Microwave Cheesecake   39
18. 18. Coconut Keto No-Bake Dessert Bars   41
19. 19. 3 Ingredient Keto Mug Cake   43
20. 20. No-Bake Keto Peanut Butter Chocolate Bars   45
21. 21. Quick Keto Chocolate Mousse   49
22. 22. Keto Pumpkin Pie   51
23. 23. Keto Chocolate Chip Cookies   53
24. 24. 5-Minute Keto Dessert   55
25. 25. No-Bake Coconut Keto Bars   57
26. 26. Creamy Keto Cheesecake Fluff   59
27. 27. Keto Chocolate Chaffee   62
28. 28. Keto Chocolate Cookies   64
29. 29. Keto Chocolate Chaffle Recipe   66
30. 30. Keto Chocolate Frosty Dessert   68

01. NO-BAKE KETO DESSERTS: PEANUT BUTTER CHOCOLATE BARS

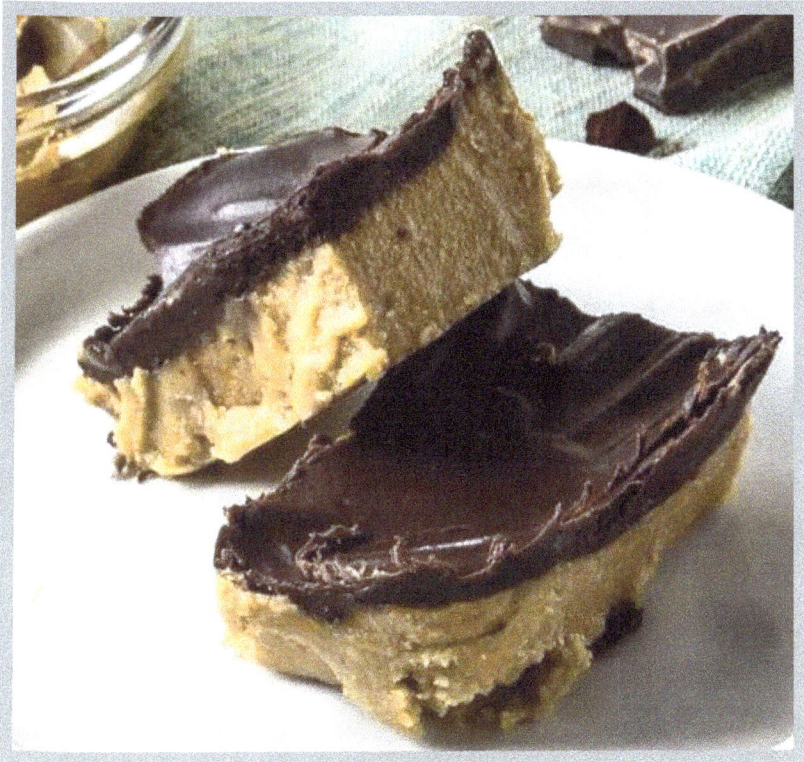

PREPARATION TIME: 2 minutes
Cooking time: 8 minutes
Ready in: 10 minutes

INGREDIENTS:

FOR THE BARS:

1. 3/4 cup (84 g) Superfine Almond Flour
    2. 2 oz (56.7 g) Butter
    3. 1/4 cup (45.5 g) Swerve, Icing sugar style
    4. 1/2 cup (129 g) Creamy Peanut Butter
    5. 1 tsp Vanilla extract

FOR THE TOPPING:

1. 1/2 cup (90 g) Sugar-Free Chocolate Chips

INSTRUCTIONS:

1. At first mix all the ingredients for the bars together and spread into a small 6-inch pan

2. Then melt the chocolate chips in a microwave oven for 30 seconds and stir.

3. Then add another 10 seconds if needed to melt fully.

4. Now spread the topping on top of the bars.

5. Final stage: refrigerate for at least an hour or two until the bars thicken up, and these bars definitely improve with keeping, so don't be in a huge rush to eat them.

02. KETO CAKE – (THE BEST CHOCOLATE RECIPE)

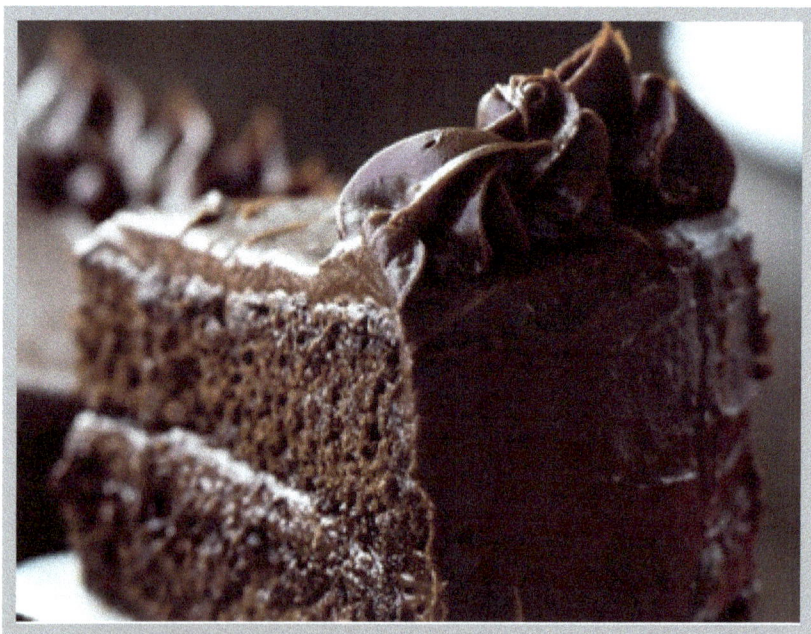

PREPARATION TIME: 5 minutes
Cooking time: 20 minutes

Ready in: 25 minutes

INGREDIENTS:

1. 1 1/2 cups fine almond flour
2. 1/4 cup cocoa powder
3. 2 tbsp Dutch cocoa or additional regular
4. 2 1/4 tsp baking powder
5. 1/2 tsp salt
6. 1/3 cup water or milk of choice
7. 3 eggs, including the vegan option listed earlier in the post
8. 1/3 cup granulated erythritol or regular sugar
9. 1 1/2 tsp pure vanilla extract

INSTRUCTIONS:

1. First stage: for a double layer cake, simply double the recipe and bake in two 8-inch pans.

2. Then preheat oven to 350 F and grease an 8-inch pan or line with parchment. Then stir all ingredients together very well, and then spread into the pan. If you needed, use the second sheet of parchment to smooth down. Then bake 16 minutes on the center rack (some ovens require more baking time, so continue cooking until firm if needed).

3. Let's cool completely before frosting.

03. LOW CARB KETO CREAM CHEESE COOKIES

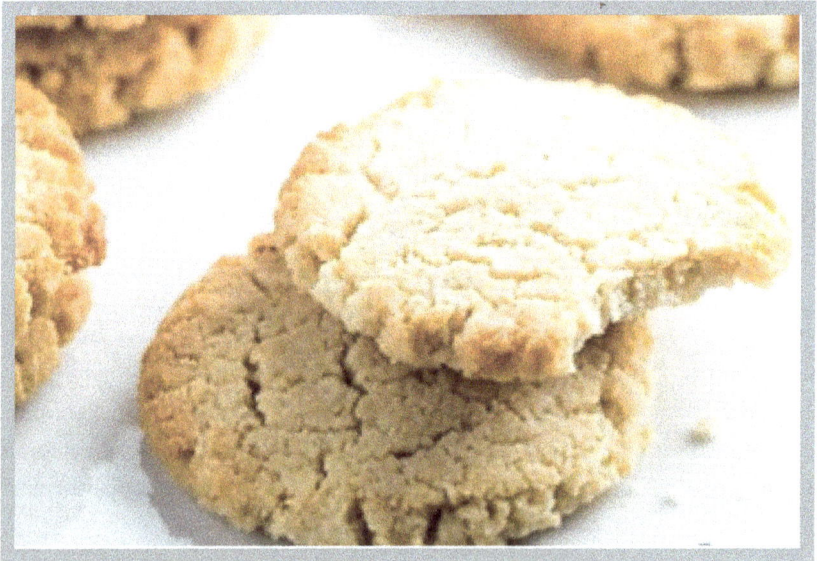

PREPARATION TIME: 10 minutes
  Cooking time: 15 minutes
  Ready in: 25 minutes

. . .

INGREDIENTS:

1. 1/4 cup Butter (softened)
2. 2 oz Cream cheese (softened)
3. 1/3 cup Monk Fruit Blend (or up to 1/2 cup if you like them very sweet)
4. 1 large Egg
5. 2 tsp Vanilla extract
6. 1/4 tsp Sea salt
7. 1 tbsp Sour cream (optional)
8. 3 cups Blanched almond flour

INSTRUCTIONS:

1. At first, preheat the oven to 350 degrees F (177 degrees C) and line a large cookie sheet with parchment paper.
2. Then use a hand mixer or stand mixer to beat together the butter, cream cheese, and sweetener until it's fluffy and light in color.
3. Do beat in the vanilla extract, salt, and egg. Beat in sour cream, if using (optional).
4. Then beat in the almond flour, 1/2 cup (64 g) at a time.
5. You can use a medium cookie scoop (about 1 1/2 tbsp, 22 mL volume) to scoop balls of the dough onto the prepared cookie sheet. Flatten with your palm.
6. Then bake for about 15mins until the edges are lightly golden. Please allow cooling completely in the pan before handling (cookies will harden as they cool).

04. KETO LEMON BARS

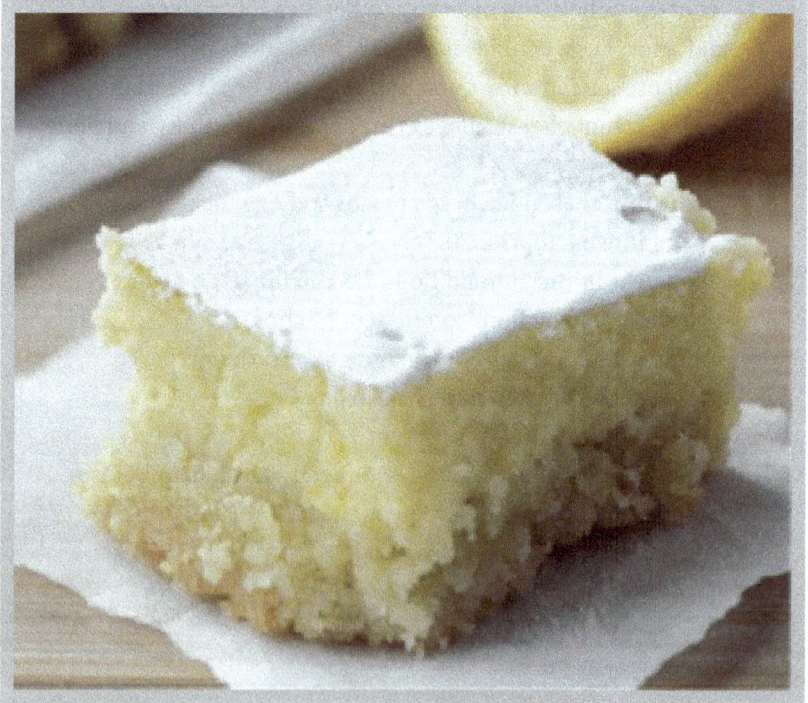

PREPARATION TIME: 15 minutes
    Cooking time: 45 minutes
    Ready in: 60 minutes

INGREDIENTS:

1. 1/2 cup butter, melted
    2. 1 3/4 cups almond flour, divided
    3. 1 cup powdered erythritol, divided
    4. 3 medium lemons
    5. 3 large eggs

INSTRUCTIONS:

1. At first mix butter, 1 cup almond flour, 1/4 cup erythritol, and a pinch of salt. Then press evenly into an 8×8″ parchment paper-lined baking dish and bake for 20 minutes at 350 degrees F. And then, let's cool for 10 minutes.

2. Then into a bowl, zest one of the lemons, juice all 3 lemons, add the eggs, 3/4 cup erythritol, 3/4 cup almond flour & pinch of salt. Now combine to make the filling.

3. Then pour the filling onto the crust & bake for 25 minutes.
    4. Final part: serve with lemon slices and a sprinkle of erythritol.

05. 3 INGREDIENT KETO CHOCOLATE COCONUT CUPS

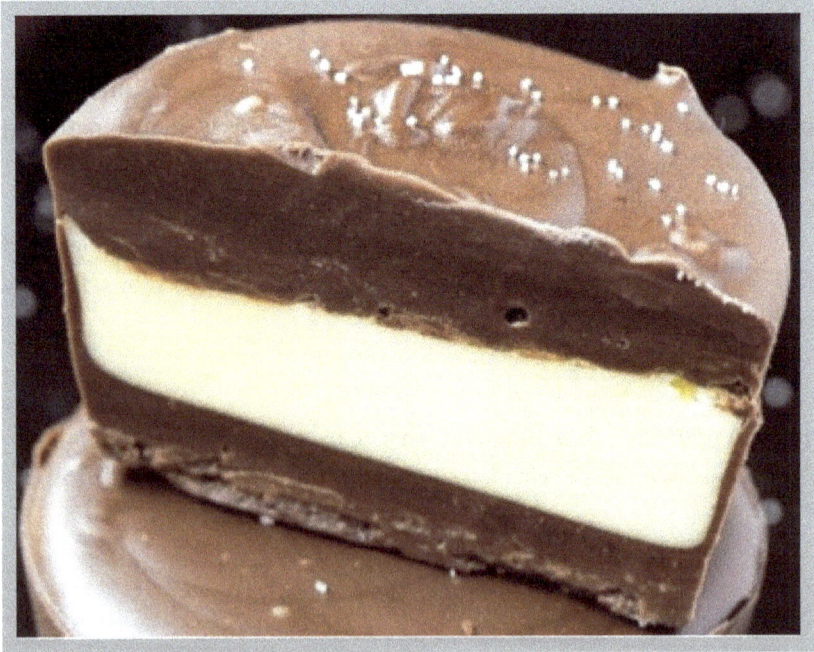

PREPARATION TIME: 2 minutes
   Cooking time: 3 minutes

Ready in: 5 minutes

INGREDIENTS:

For the keto version

1. 1/2 cup coconut butter, melted
   2. 1/2 cup cocoa powder
   3. 1/2 cup coconut oil
   4. 1 serving sweetener of choice See notes

FOR THE NON-KETO version

1. 1 cup chocolate chips of choice
   2. 1/2 cup coconut butter, melted

INSTRUCTIONS:

1. At first, line an 18-count mini muffin tin with mini muffin liners and set aside.

2. Then in a microwave-safe bowl or stovetop, melt your coconut oil and add your cocoa powder and mix until fully combined and no clumps remain. If you want to use options to add a sweetener, add it here now too.

3. Now moving quickly, coat the bottom and sides of the muffin liners with melted chocolate and ensure a little is leftover to top with water. Now place the chocolate-coated muffin tins in the freezer to firm up.

. . .

4. Final stage: once firm, divide the coconut butter amongst the cups and top with the remaining chocolate and freeze until firm.

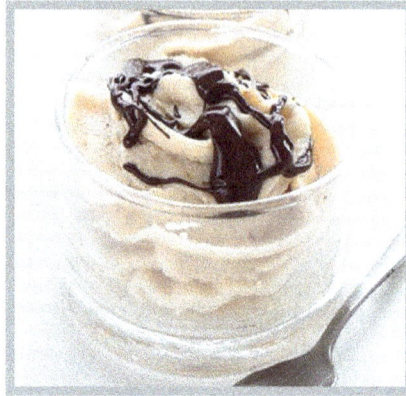

PREPARATION TIME: 2 minutes
   Cooking time: 3 minutes
   Ready in: 5 minutes

INGREDIENTS:

1. ½ cup heavy whipping cream (more if needed to thin the mixture)
   2. 4 oz cream cheese (softened)
   3. 1/4 cup natural peanut butter (no sugar added)
   4. 1/4 cup powdered Swerve Sweetener
   5. ½ tsp vanilla extract

INSTRUCTIONS:

. . .

1. Take a medium bowl; whip the 1/2 cup of cream until it holds stiff peaks.

2. Then in another medium bowl, beat together the cream cheese and peanut butter until smooth and creamy and add the sweetener and vanilla. If your peanut butter looks unsalted, then add a pinch of salt as well. Do beat until smooth.

3. Now, if your mixture is overly thick, add about 2 tbsp heavy cream to lighten it and beat until combined.

4. Then gently fold in the whipped cream until no streaks remain and spoon or pipe into little dessert glasses.

5. Final stage: drizzle with a little low carb chocolate sauce, if desired.

06. PEANUT BUTTER MOUSSE – KETO AND SUGAR-FREE

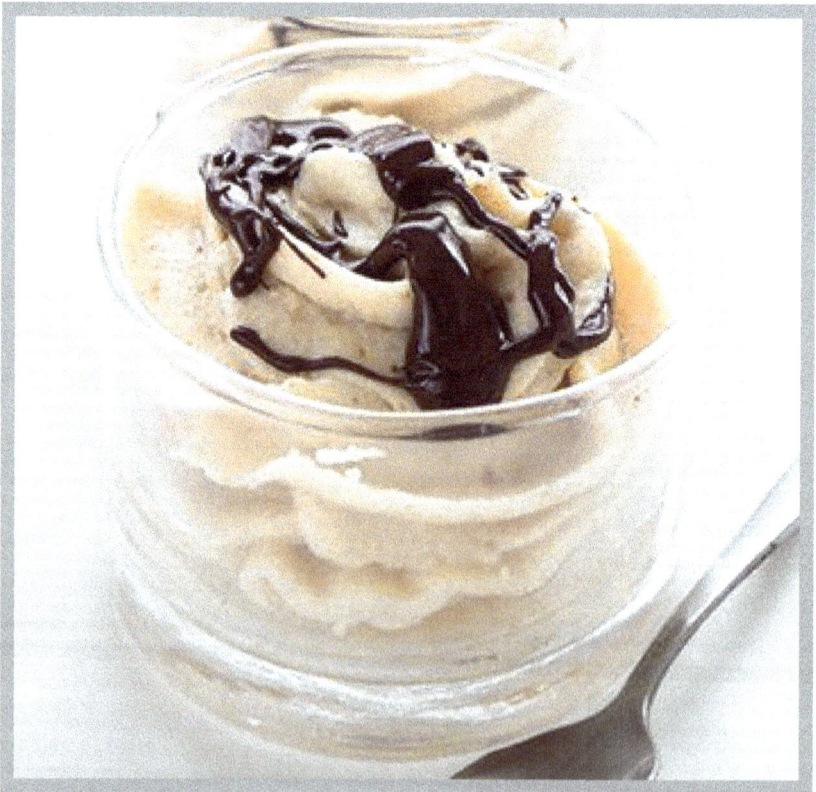

PREPARATION TIME: 2 minutes
  Cooking time: 3 minutes
  Ready in: 5 minutes

INGREDIENTS:

1. ½ cup heavy whipping cream (more if needed to thin the mixture)
   2. 4 oz cream cheese (softened)
   3. 1/4 cup natural peanut butter (no sugar added)
   4. 1/4 cup powdered Swerve Sweetener
   5. ½ tsp vanilla extract

INSTRUCTIONS:

1. Take a medium bowl; whip the 1/2 cup of cream until it holds stiff peaks.

2. Then in another medium bowl, beat together the cream cheese and peanut butter until smooth and creamy and add the sweetener and vanilla. If your peanut butter looks unsalted, then add a pinch of salt as well. Do beat until smooth.

3. Now, if your mixture is overly thick, add about 2 tbsp heavy cream to lighten it and beat until combined.

4. Then gently fold in the whipped cream until no streaks remain and spoon or pipe into little dessert glasses.

5. Final stage: drizzle with a little low carb chocolate sauce, if desired.

Chapter Seven

07. KETO NO-BAKE COOKIES

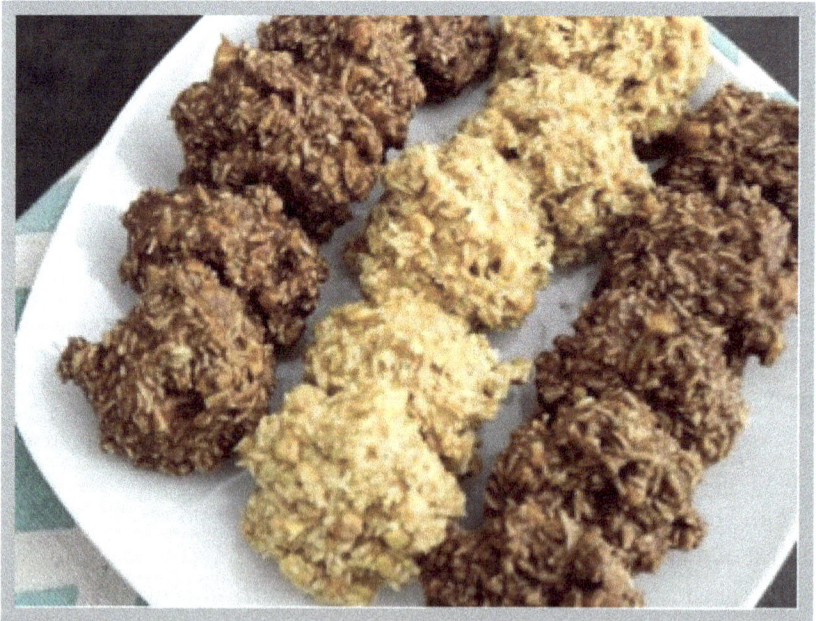

PREPARATION TIME: 2 minutes
Cooking time: 3 minutes

Ready in: 5 minutes

INGREDIENTS:

1. 2 tablespoons real butter
    2. 2/3 cup all-natural peanut butter, or your choice of nut butter

3. 1 cup unsweetened all-natural shredded coconut

4. 4 drops of vanilla,

INSTRUCTIONS:

1. At first, melt butter in microwave.

2. Then stir in peanut butter.
    3. Plus, sweetener and coconut and mix well.

4. Now spoon onto a sheet pan.

5. Then freeze for 5-10 minutes.
    6. Final stage: store in the refrigerator, bagged.

08. KETO CHOCOLATE CHIP COOKIES

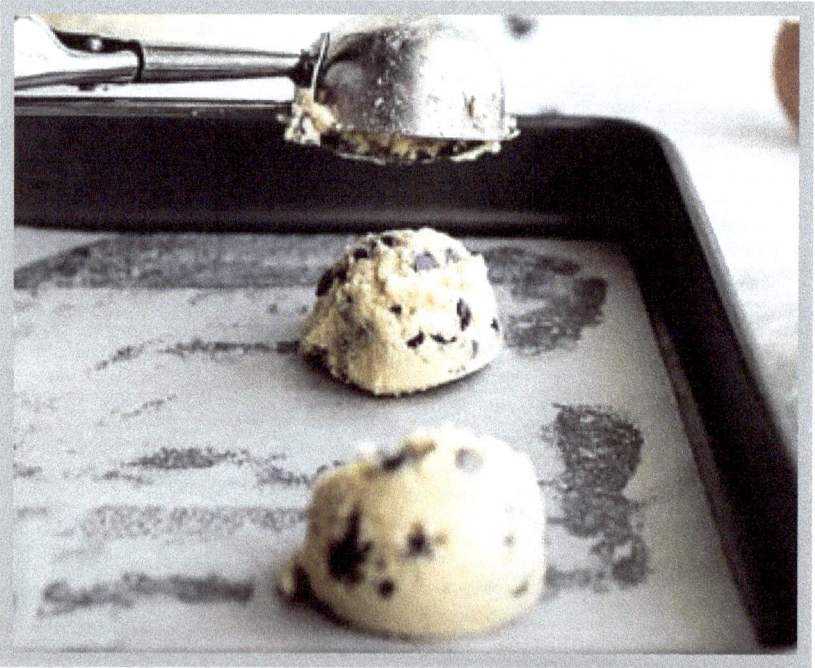

PREPARATION TIME: 10 minutes
Cooking time: 20 minutes
Ready in: 50 minutes

INGREDIENTS:

1. 3.5 oz Salted Butter (3.5 oz - 1/2 cup)
2. 4.5 oz Erythritol (4.5 oz - 3/4 cup)
3. 1 tsp Vanilla Extract
4. 1 large Egg (50g / 1.7 oz)
5. 6 oz Almond Flour (6 oz - 1 1/2 cups)
6. 1/2 tsp baking powder
7. 1/2 tsp xanthan gum (optional)
8. 1/4 tsp Salt
9. 3 oz Sugar-Free Chocolate Chips (30g - 3/4 cup)

INSTRUCTIONS:

1. At first, preheat the oven to 180C (355F). Then microwave the butter for 30 seconds to melt, but make sure it is not hot.

2. Then place the butter and erythritol in a mixing bowl and beat until combined and add the vanilla and egg, and beat on low for another 15 seconds exactly.

3. Plus, the almond flour, baking powder, xanthan gum, and salt and beat until well combined.

4. Please press the dough together and remove it from the bowl.

. . .

5. Then divide and shape the dough into 12 balls (or use a small ice cream scoop) and place it on a baking tray. Do bake for 10 minutes at 180C (355F).

6. Final round: allow to cool before serving. Keep in an airtight container for up to 7 days.

09. KETO CHEESECAKE BROWNIES

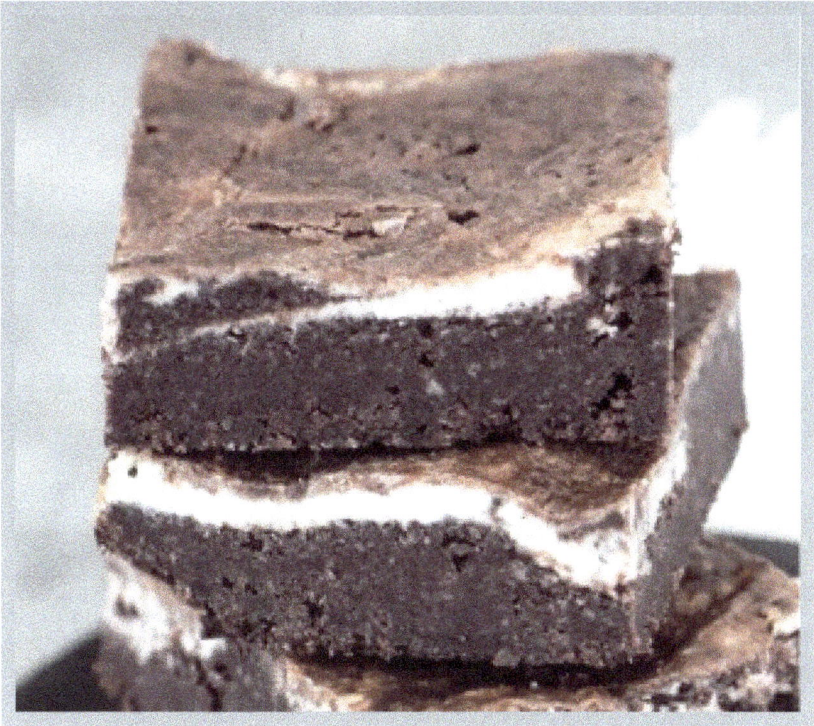

PREPARATION TIME: 10 minutes
  Cooking time: 25 minutes
  Ready in: 35 minutes

INGREDIENTS:

FOR THE BROWNIES:
  1. 8 tablespoons butter, melted
  2. 3/4 cup Swerve granulated sugar substitute. (Erythritol only, no substitutions)
  3. 1/3 cup unsweetened cocoa powder
  4. 2 eggs, beaten
  5. 1/2 teaspoon salt
  6. 3/4 cup almond flour
  7. For the cheesecake layer:
  8. 4 ounces softened cream cheese
  9. 3 tablespoon swerve sweetener (confectioners best here instead of granulated, but granulated will work if it is all you have)
  10. 2 tablespoons heavy cream
  11. 2 teaspoons vanilla extract

INSTRUCTIONS:

  1. First, preheat oven to 350 degrees.
  2. Then line an 8x8 baking pan with parchment paper and set aside.
  3. Take a mixing bowl, combine the melted butter, Swerve sugar substitute, and cocoa powder until completely combined.
  4. Then mix in the eggs, stir well.
  5. Now add the almond flour and salt, stir well and spread the brownie mixture to all four corners of your baking pan, set aside.

6. Now in a blender or food processor, add the cream cheese, swerve sugar substitute, heavy cream, and vanilla extract and blend for 15 seconds, scrape down the edges and blend again.
7. Then spoon the cheesecake mixture in lumps onto the brownie batter, and swirl.
8. Now both the brownie and the cheesecake layer are quite thick, they will probably not create beautiful "swirls," but the thickness does create great layers of sweet cheesecake and fuggy brownie.
9. Do bake for 25-30 minutes or until brownies are set
10. Final stage: allow to cool and slice, store in the refrigerator.

10. BEST EVER KETO CHOCOLATE CAKE

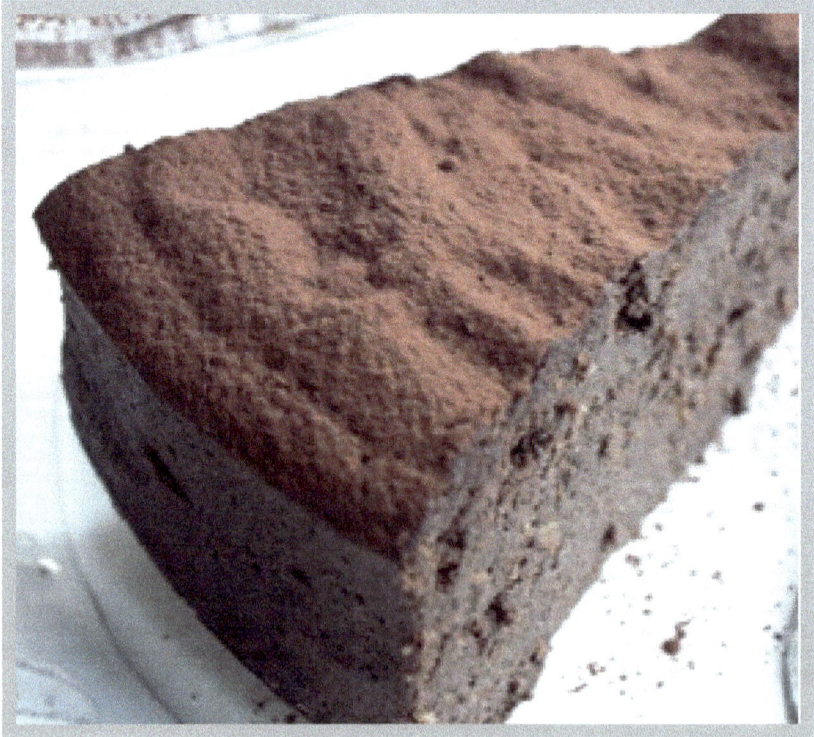

PREPARATION TIME: 10 minutes
 Cooking time: 30 minutes
 Ready in: 40 minutes

INGREDIENTS:

1. 300 g / 10.5 oz unsweetened chocolate
2. 300 g / 10.5 oz butter unsalted (1 1/3 cup melted)
3. 6 eggs
4. 1/2 cup / 50g almond flour or ground almonds
5. 1 cup / 150g powdered erythritol
6. Pinch of salt

INSTRUCTIONS:

1. at first, heat the oven to 170 Celsius / 340 Fahrenheit. (If you are baking at high altitude, increase the oven temperature by 10 Celsius / 25 Fahrenheit.)

2. Then melt the butter and chocolate in the microwave (ca 90 seconds), then stir and wait until dissolved. Alternatively, gently heat in a water bath.

3. Take a large bowl, beat the eggs until foamy, then add the sweetener and mix well.

4. Then add the melted chocolate and butter along with the almond flour and stir with a spoon or spatula until just combined.

5. Now line the bottom of a 20 cm / 8-inch springform with parchment paper and grease the sides with butter and pour in the cake batter and bake for 25 mins on the middle shelf until the top of the cake is firm to the touch.

6. Final stage: leave to cool before releasing from the cake tin. When the cake is completely cooled, dust with cocoa powder.

11. NUT-FREE KETO BROWNIE

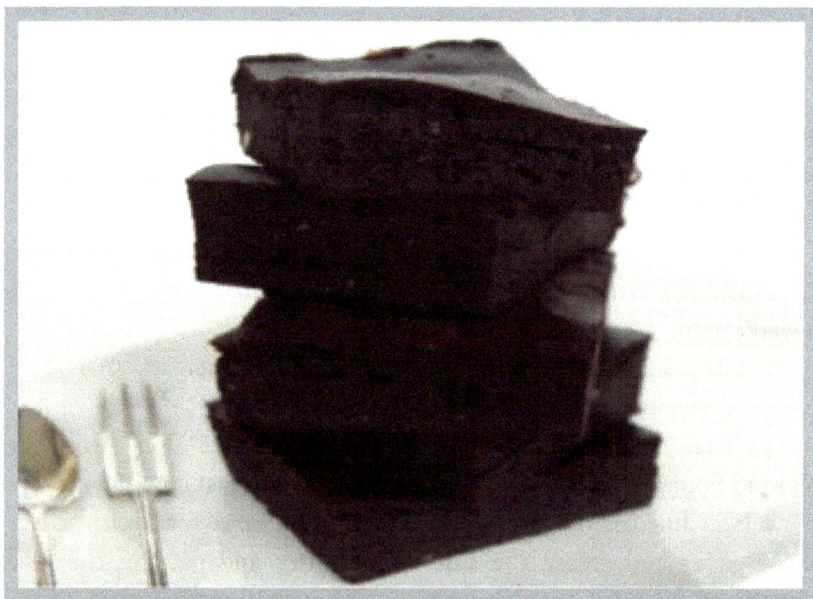

PREPARATION TIME: 10 minutes
   Cooking time: 20 minutes
   Ready in: 30 minutes

Ingredients:

1. 6 eggs - medium
2. 160 g butter melted
3. 60 g cocoa unsweetened
4. 1/2 tsp baking powder
5. 2 tsp vanilla
6. 120 g cream cheese softened
7. 4 tbsp granulated sweetener of choice or more, to your taste

Instructions:

1. At first, place all the ingredients in a mixing bowl and using a stick blender with the blade attachment, blend until smooth.

2. Then pour into a lined square baking dish (21cm/8.5 inch).

3. Do bake at 180C/350F for 20-25 minutes until cooked in the center.

4. Final stage: slice into squares, rectangle bars, or triangle wedges.

12. EASY KETO CHOCOLATE FROSTY

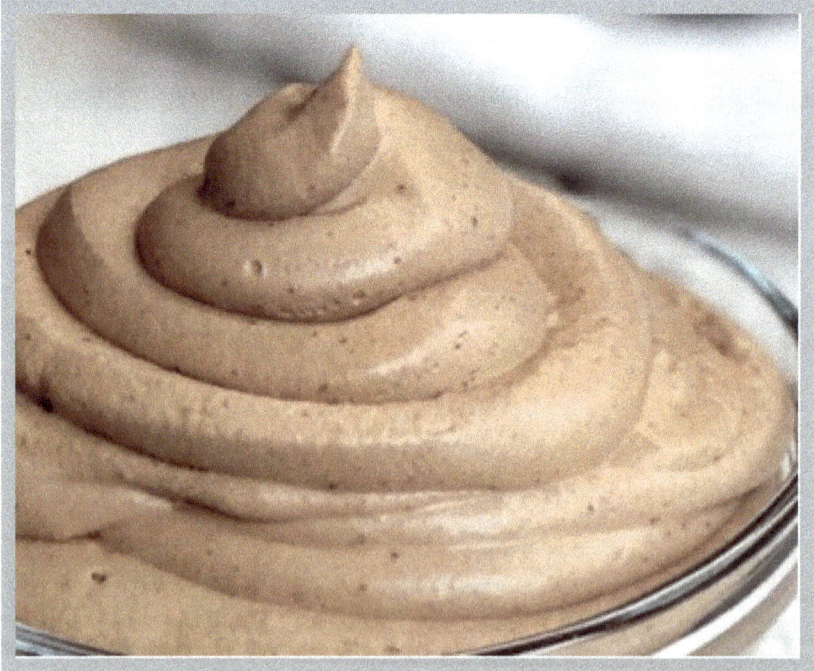

PREPARATION TIME: **5 minutes**

Cooking time: 30 minutes
Ready in: 35 minutes

INGREDIENTS:

1. 1 cup heavy whipping cream
    2. 2 tbsp unsweetened cocoa powder
    3. 1 tbsp almond butter
    4. 1 tsp vanilla extract
    5. 5 drops liquid stevia (or sweetener of your choice)

INSTRUCTIONS:

1. At first, take a medium-size bowl, use a hand mixer to beat the heavy cream for a few minutes.

2. Then add the rest of the ingredients and blend again until the mixture becomes the consistency of thick whipped cream or frosting.

3. Final stage: place in the freezer for about 30 minutes or until it's the consistency you like.
    4. Enjoy!

Chapter Thirteen

13. EASY KETO MUFFINS

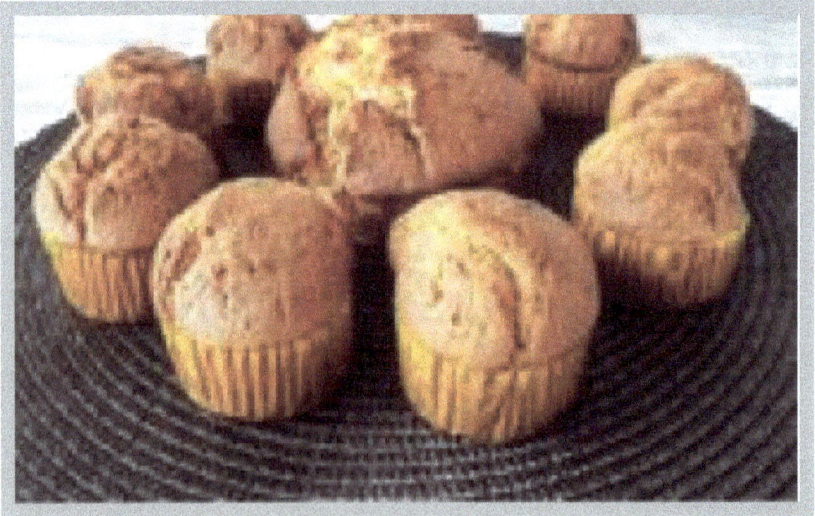

PREPARATION TIME: 5 minutes
   Cooking time: 15 minutes
   Ready in: 20 minutes

. . .

INGREDIENTS:

1. 3 cups almond flour
    2. 1/2 cup Unsalted Butter melted (but not hot)
    3. 4 large eggs
    4. 1 Orange zest and juice
    5. 1 tsp baking soda
    6. Stevia syrup or other sweeteners to taste

INSTRUCTIONS:

1. At first, preheat the oven to 350.° F or 175.° C.

2. Then mix all ingredients in a large mixing bowl and add stevia to taste.

3. Final stage: pour into muffins pan and bake for 15 - 20 minutes.

Chapter Fourteen

14. NO-BAKE KETO CHOCOLATE CHIP COOKIE BARS

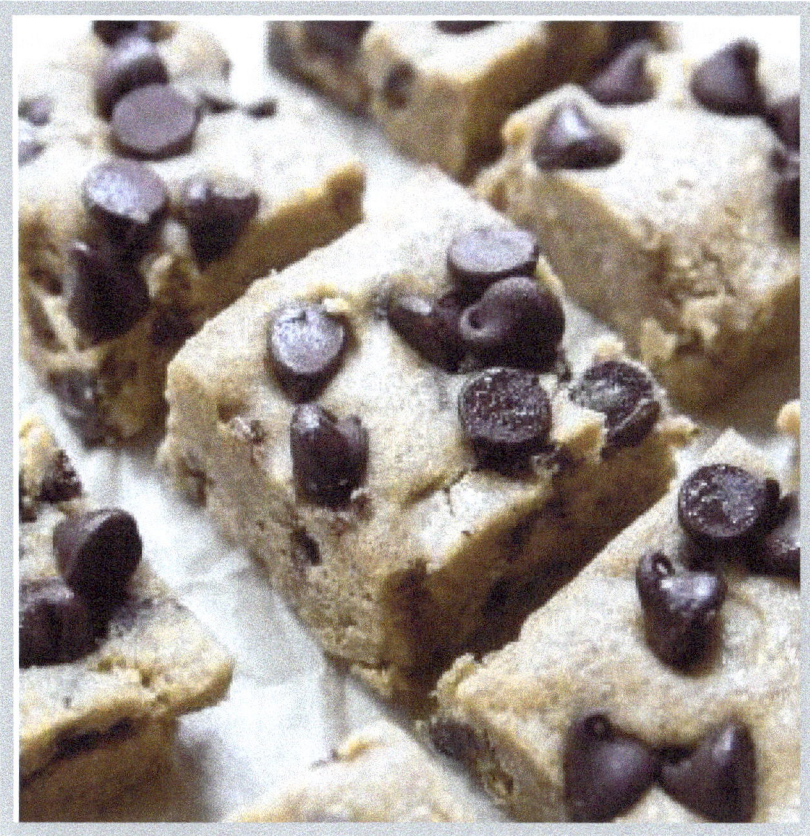

PREPARATION TIME: 5 minutes
   Cooking time: 60 minutes
   Ready in: 65 minutes

INGREDIENTS:
   1. 1 cup almond flour
   2. 1/2 cup almond butter
   3. 1/4 cup ghee
   4. 1/2 cup confectioners sugar-free sweetener
   5. 1/2 cup sugar-free chocolate chips

. . .

Optional Add-ins:

1. 1 tsp pure vanilla extract
2. 1/2 tsp ground cinnamon
3. 1/4 tsp sea salt

Instructions:

1. At first, add the almond butter and ghee to a mixing bowl and microwave it for 20 to 30 seconds, or until softened. You have to want these ingredients to be very soft (or melted) so that they stir easily.
2. Then add the remaining ingredients except for the chocolate chips to the mixing bowl and stir until well-combined. When the dough is well-mixed, fold in the chocolate chips.
3. Then transfer the cookie dough to a parchment-lined loaf pan (mine is 9" x 5") and freeze for 1 hour. Once you're ready to serve, thaw, and then use a sharp knife to cut squares.
4. Then store leftovers in the refrigerator or freezer in a sealed container or bag.

15. LOW CARB LEMON MOUSSE RECIPE

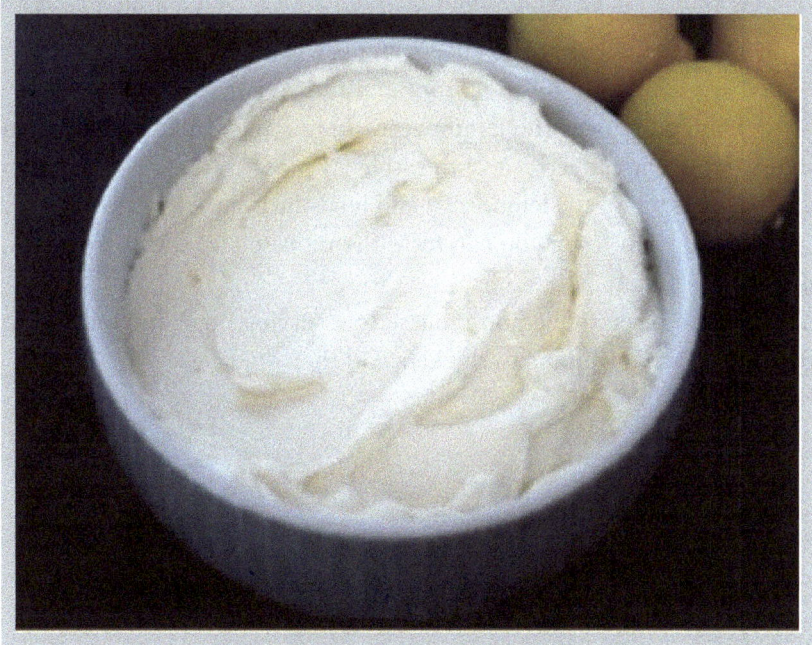

PREPARATION TIME: **5 minutes**
   Cooking time: **5 minutes**

Ready in: 10 minutes

INGREDIENTS:

1. 1 Cup Cream (Heavy, Double or Whipping)
    2. 1/2 Cup Cream Cheese, softened
    3. 2-4 Tablespoons Stevia
    4. 1/2 to 1 Lemon – juice and zest

INSTRUCTIONS:

1. At first, pour the cream into a large bowl.

    2. When using an electric beater, whip the cream until thickened.

    3. Then add in the cream cheese and stevia.

    4. Now whip until fully incorporated and creamy.

    5. Then grate over the lemon zest, using a micro-plane grater, and squeeze the lemon over a sieve to catch any pips.

    6. Now whip in the lemon zest and juice until smooth.

    7. If you want, then you can taste the mousse and add more stevia, if needed.

    8. Please place the lemon mousse to a serving bowl and move into the fridge for a few hours to thicken, and then enjoy.

16. KETO CHOCOLATE CHEESECAKE BITES

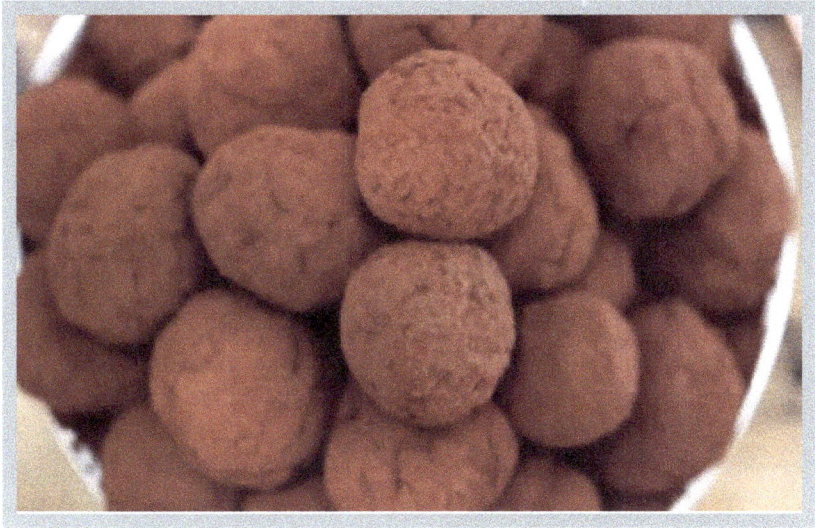

PREPARATION TIME: 30 minutes
  Cooking time: 30 minutes
  Ready in: 60 minutes

. . .

INGREDIENTS:

1. 3.4 ounces package low-carb/sugar-free instant chocolate pudding
2. 8 ounces cream cheese (room temperature)
3. 1 teaspoon vanilla extract
4. 1/4 teaspoon salt
5. 1/3 cup Powdered Erythritol Sweetener (or Powdered Swerve Sweetener)
6. 1/3 cup unsweetened cocoa powder

INSTRUCTIONS:

1. Take a medium bowl, mix the chocolate pudding, cream cheese, vanilla, salt, powdered sugar.
2. Then chill the mixture for 30 minutes.
3. And add cocoa powder to a small bowl.
4. Now use a 1 tablespoon cookie scoop to form the dough into balls then dip in a small bowl of cocoa powder until coated.
5. Final stage: chill for 30 minutes and enjoy!

17. KETO MICROWAVE CHEESECAKE

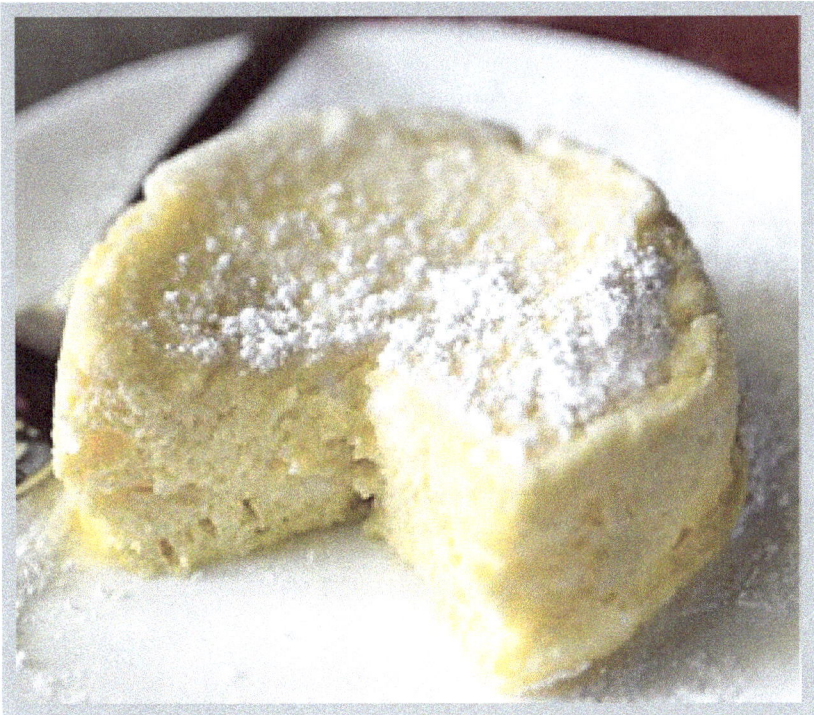

PREPARATION TIME: 5 minutes
   Cooking time: 12 minutes
   Ready in: 17 minutes

INGREDIENTS:

1. 2 oz Neufchatel cream cheese, cubed
   2. 1/4 teaspoon pure vanilla extract
   3. 1/2 teaspoon stevia glycerite (equals about 2 tablespoons sugar)
   4. 1 large egg

INSTRUCTIONS:

1. At first place, the cream cheese in a 1-cup, 3-inch wide ceramic ramekin and microwave 15 seconds to soften.

2. Then add the vanilla and stevia and mix with a fork to combine.
   3. Do mix in the egg, patiently and thoroughly, until smooth. This process will take a couple of minutes.
   4. Then do microwave for 90 seconds.
   5. Now allow the cake to rest and cool in the ramekin for 10 minutes, then run a knife around the edges and carefully invert it onto a plate.
   6. Final stage: top with your choice of toppings and serve, or refrigerate until ready to serve and remove from fridge 15 minutes before serving.

18. COCONUT KETO NO-BAKE DESSERT BARS

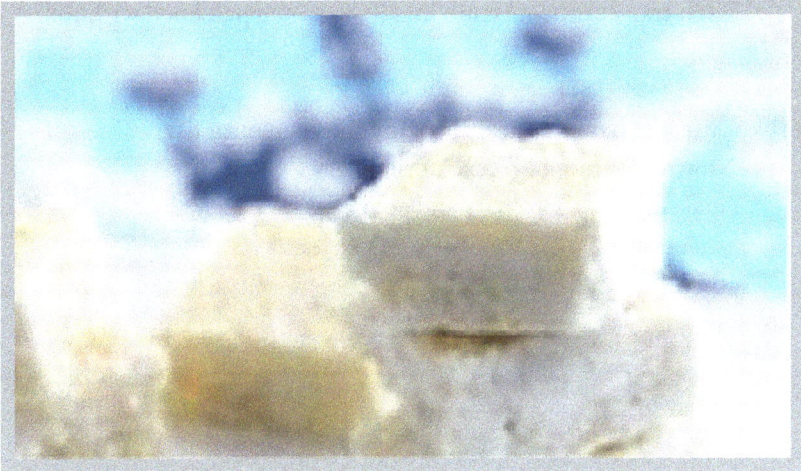

PREPARATION TIME: 1 hour
   Cooking time: 2 hours
   Ready in: 3 hours

INGREDIENTS:

. . .

1. 3 cups unsweetened coconut shreds
    2. 1 cup coconut oil
    3. 3-4 Tbsp low-carb fiber syrup (or liquid sweetener of choice, honey, maple syrup, etc.)
    4. ½ tsp vanilla extract
    5. Pinch of salt

INSTRUCTIONS:

1. First time take a large mixing bowl; mix everything until you have a thick mixture. If you feel it's crumbly, add a bit of extra fiber syrup or the liquid sweetener of your choice.
    2. Then transfer the mixture into an 8×8-inch pan lined with foil.

3. Now use wet hands to press mixture into pan until flat.
    4. Now refrigerate or freeze until firm.
    5. Final stage: cut into bars and enjoy!

19. 3 INGREDIENT KETO MUG CAKE

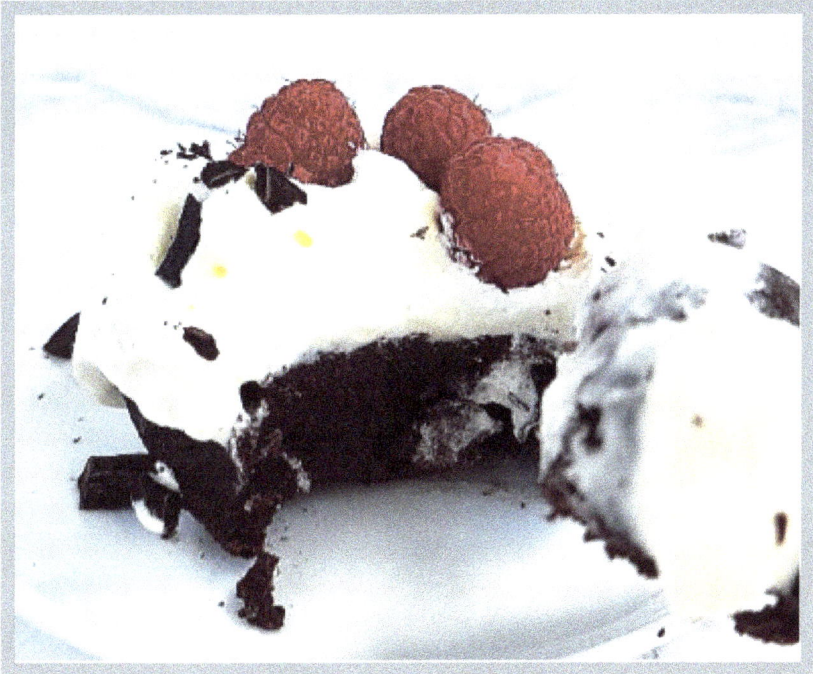

PREPARATION TIME: **2 minutes**

Cooking time: 2 minutes
Ready in: 4 minutes

INGREDIENTS:

1. 1 egg
    2. 2 tbsp Erythritol (or another sweetener of your choice)
    3. 2 tbsp cacao powder

INSTRUCTIONS:

1. At first, whisk all the ingredients together in a small bowl or a mug.

2. Then pour the mix into a greased microwave-safe ramekin or a mug.
    3. Now microwave for 60 seconds.
    4. Final stage: serve immediately, this low carb chocolate cake in a mug tastes best right after you make it, if you leave it for too long it can turn spongey.

Chapter Twenty

20. NO-BAKE KETO PEANUT BUTTER CHOCOLATE BARS

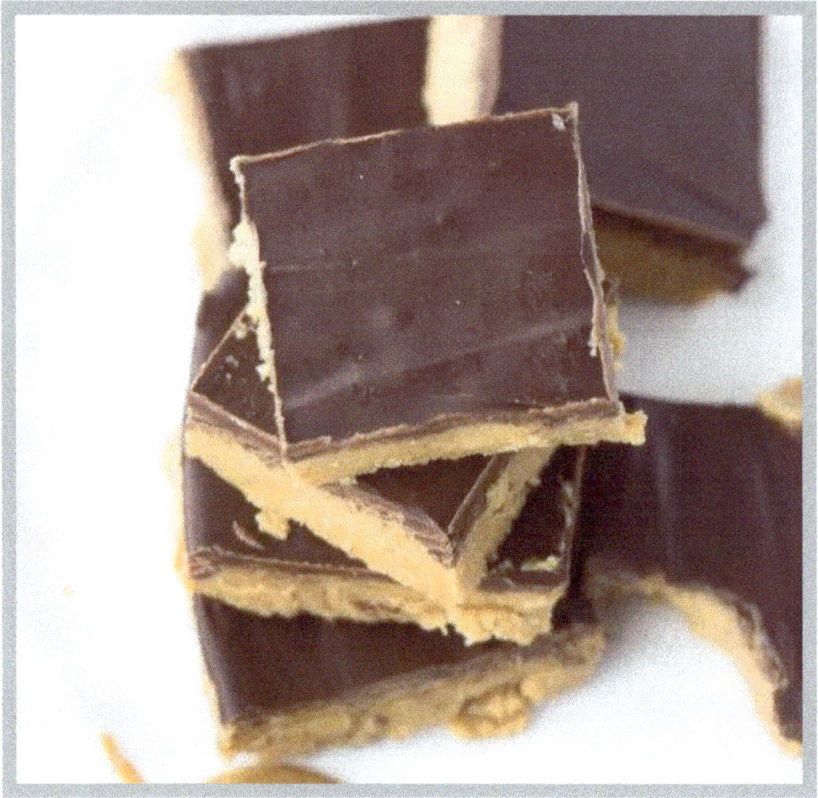

PREPARATION TIME: 5 minutes
   Cooking time: 120 minutes
   Ready in: 125 minutes

INGREDIENTS:

1. 1 cup Natural Peanut Butter
   2. 4 tbsp butter, softened
   3. 2/3 cup Powdered Monk fruit

4. 2 tbsp coconut flour

FOR THE CHOCOLATE TOPPING:

1. 1 tbsp butter
2. 1 3oz Chocolate Candy Bar

INSTRUCTIONS

1. At first, take a bowl, beat the softened butter at high speed.

2.THEN add powdered Monk fruit powdered, peanut butter, and coconut then beat with a mixer again on medium until all of the ingredients are thoroughly combined.

3. Now line a 9 X 9-inch baking pan with parchment paper (or grease pan) and spread the peanut butter layer evenly then place in the freezer for 10 minutes.

4. Then meanwhile, tear the Lily's Smooth Creamy Chocolate Bar into pieces in a small greased glass container and add 1 tablespoon of butter.

5. Do microwave for 30 seconds, and then stir. If you see, it is not completely melted microwave in 15-second intervals stirring between until it is and make sure always to stir as it will continue to melt when you stir it. Please do not overcook, or the chocolate will become hard and will not spread.

6. Please remove the baking pan from the freezer and spread the pour the chocolate layer on top of the peanut butter layer, then using a spatula spread it evenly.

· · ·

7. Final stage: return to the freezer for several hours or overnight to allow the No-Bake Keto Peanut Butter Bars to setup. When they have set up, you can store either in the freezer or the fridge.

21. QUICK KETO CHOCOLATE MOUSSE

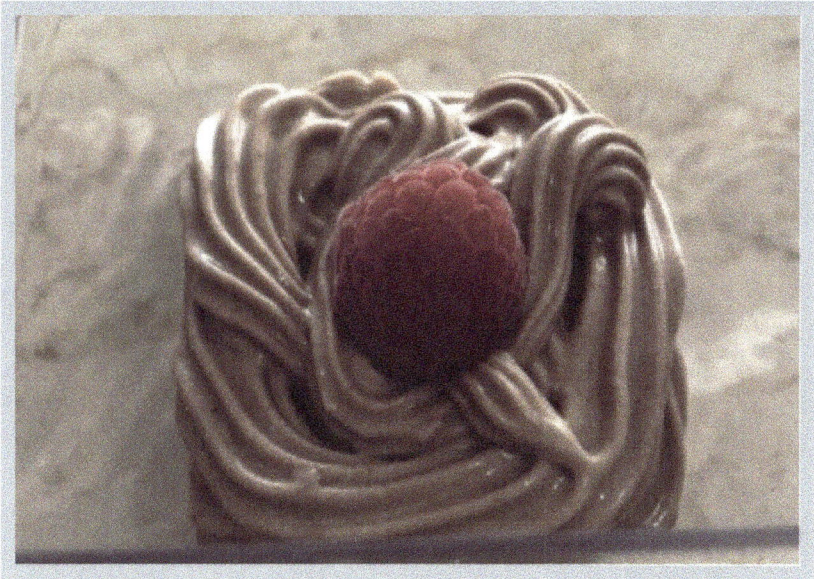

PREPARATION TIME: **2 minutes**
   Cooking time: 8 minutes
   Ready in: 10 minutes

· · ·

INGREDIENTS:

1. 3 ounces cream cheese
2. ½ cup heavy cream
3. 1 teaspoon vanilla extract
4. ¼ cup powdered zero-calorie sweeteners

5. 2 tablespoons of cocoa powder

6. 1 pinch salt

INSTRUCTIONS:

1. At first, place cream cheese in a large bowl and beat using an electric mixer until light and fluffy.

2. Then turn the mixer to low speed and slowly add heavy cream and vanilla extract and add sweetener, cocoa powder, and salt, mixing until well incorporated.

3. Now turn the mixer to high and mix until light and fluffy, 1 to 2 minutes more.

4. Final stage: serve immediately, or refrigerate for later.

22. KETO PUMPKIN PIE

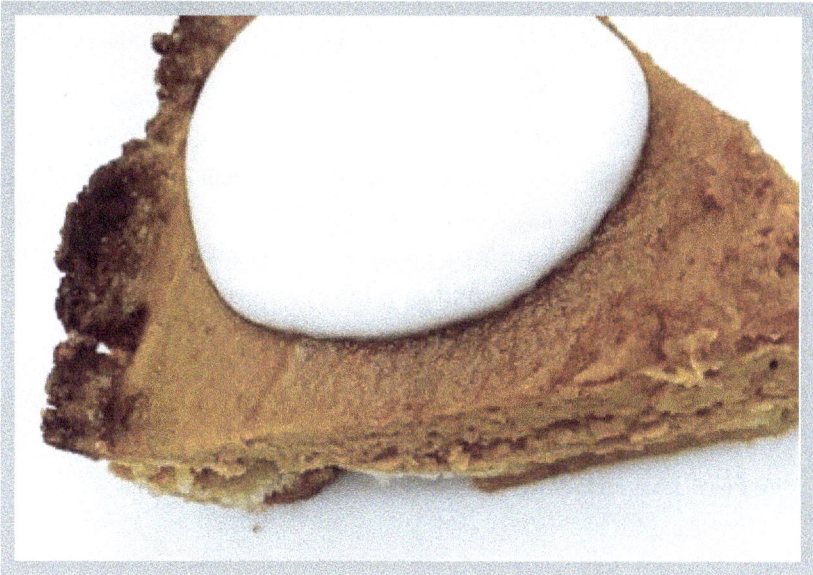

PREPARATION TIME: 10 minutes
  Cooking time: 50 minutes
  Ready in: 60 minutes

. . .

INGREDIENTS:

1. 1 almond flour pie crust
    2. 1/2 cup heavy whipping cream
    3. 1 15-oz cans pumpkin puree
    4. 2 large eggs
    5. 2/3 cup powdered erythritol.
    6. 2 tsp pumpkin pie spice or Gingerbread spice
    7. 1 tsp Vanilla extract
    8. 1/4 tsp sea salt

INSTRUCTIONS:

1. At first, make your favorite Almond Flour Pie Crust.

2. Do mix all of the ingredients together with a blender or hand mixer.

3. When the pie crust is cool, transfer the keto pumpkin pie filling into the crust. Please be careful not to overfill it!

4. Do bake at 325 for 40-50 minutes, and you want the pie to be almost set; a little soft in the middle is best to prevent cracking.

5. Please lets the pie cool at room temp or for at least an hour in the fridge before serving.

6. Final stage: top with Keto Whipping Cream and enjoy!

Chapter Twenty-Three

23. KETO CHOCOLATE CHIP COOKIES

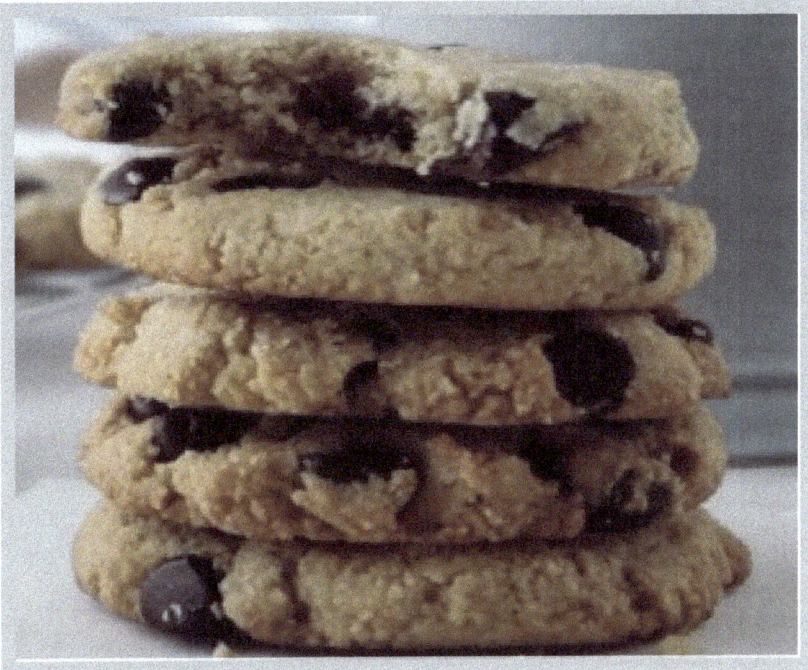

PREPARATION TIME: **5 minutes**

Cooking time: 10 minutes
Ready in: 15 minutes

INGREDIENTS:

1. 1 cup finely ground almond flour
    2. 1/4 cup Lilly's sugar-free chocolate chips

3. 2 tbsp powdered erythritol
    4. 1/4 tsp salt
    5. 1/8 tsp baking soda
    6. 2 tbsp melted butter
    7. 1 tsp pure vanilla extract
    8. 1-2 Tablespoons almond milk Optional

INSTRUCTIONS:

1. At first, preheat oven to 325 F.

2. Then stir dry ingredients very well (so you don't end up biting into a clump of baking soda!).

3. Now add wet to form a dough.

4. You can use a cookie scoop or tablespoon to form cookies.

5. Please place on a cookie tray, and bake on the center rack 10-12 minutes.

6. The last stage: lets cool an additional 10 minutes before handling, as they are very delicate at first but firm up completely once cool.

24. 5-MINUTE KETO DESSERT

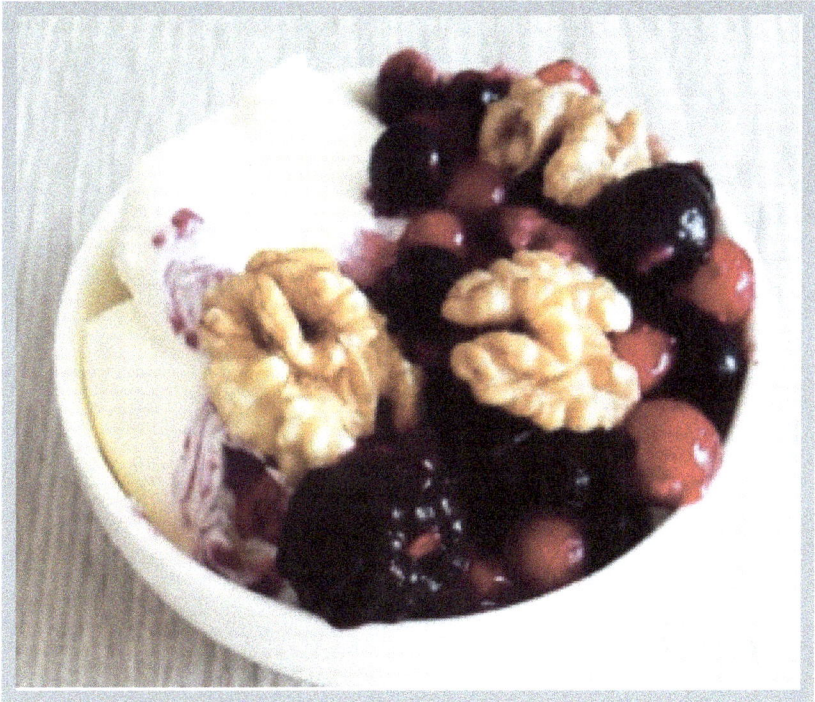

PREPARATION TIME: 1 minute
    Cooking time: 4 minutes
    Ready in: 5 minutes

INGREDIENTS:

1. 1/3 cup mascarpone
    2. 1/3 cup berries
    3. 3-4 walnut halves

INSTRUCTIONS:

1. Take a small jar, add the mascarpone, top with berries (used frozen as they weren't in season yet), and the walnuts (you can chop them if you want)! Now add stevia if needed (I didn't use any)

2. Enjoy immediately!

Chapter Twenty-Five

25. NO-BAKE COCONUT KETO BARS

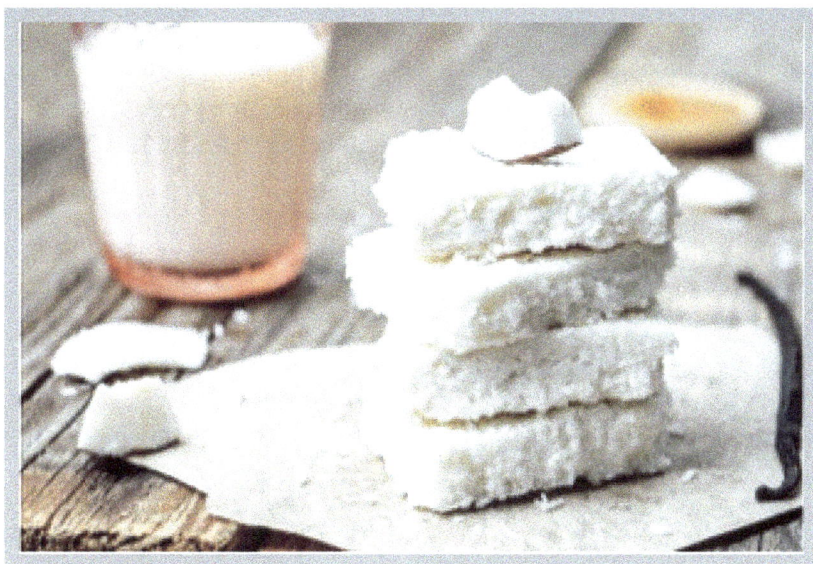

PREPARATION TIME: 5 minute
   Cooking time: 20 minutes
   Ready in: 25 minutes

. . .

INGREDIENTS:

1. 2 scoops Optimum Nutrition Unflavored 100% Plant Protein
    2. 3 cups unsweetened shredded coconut
    3. 1 cup + 2 Tbsp.Organic Coconut Oil with Butter Flavor
    4. ¼ cup + 2 Tbsp. monk fruit
    5. ¼ cup Macadamia Milk
    6. ¼ cup water
    7. 1 tsp. vanilla extract
    8. Dash Redmond Real Salt Sea Salt

INSTRUCTIONS:

1. at first line baking pan with parchment paper.
    2. Take mixing bowl; mix all ingredients until well combined.
    3. Then transfer mixture to prepared pan and press down.
    4. Final stage: chill in the fridge for 20 minutes. Cut into 12 bars.

26. CREAMY KETO CHEESECAKE FLUFF

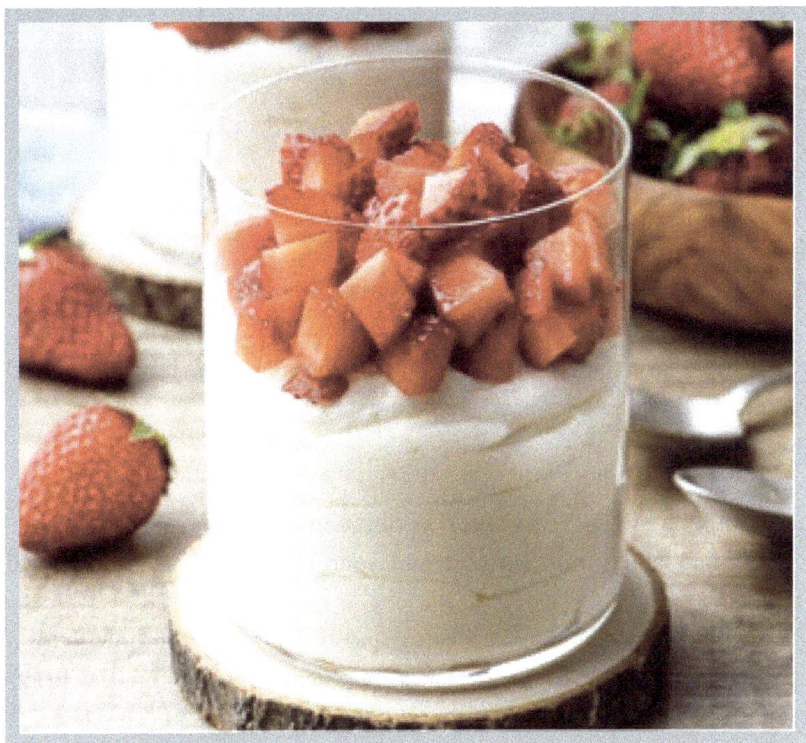

PREPARATION TIME: 5 minute
Cooking time: 10 minutes
Ready in: 15 minutes

INGREDIENTS:

1. 8 oz cream cheese
    2. 4 oz cold heavy cream
    3. 4 tbsp sour cream
    4. ¼ cup granulated stevia or another low carb granulated sweetener

5. 1 ½ tsp vanilla extract

FOR DECORATION:
    1. 1/3 cup chopped strawberries (optional)

INSTRUCTIONS:

1. At first, place the cream cheese and sweetener in the bowl of a stand mixer fitted with a paddle attachment.

2. Do mix on medium-low speed until the mixture is creamy.
    3. Then add vanilla extract and sour cream and beat until well blended.
    4. Now scrape down the beater, and the sides of the bowl with a spatula then switch to the whisk attachment and pour in the heavy cream.

. . .

5. Now whip until the mixture can hold stiff peaks.

6. Final stage: divide the mixture between the glasses, top with chopped strawberries (if using) and serve.

27. KETO CHOCOLATE CHAFFEE

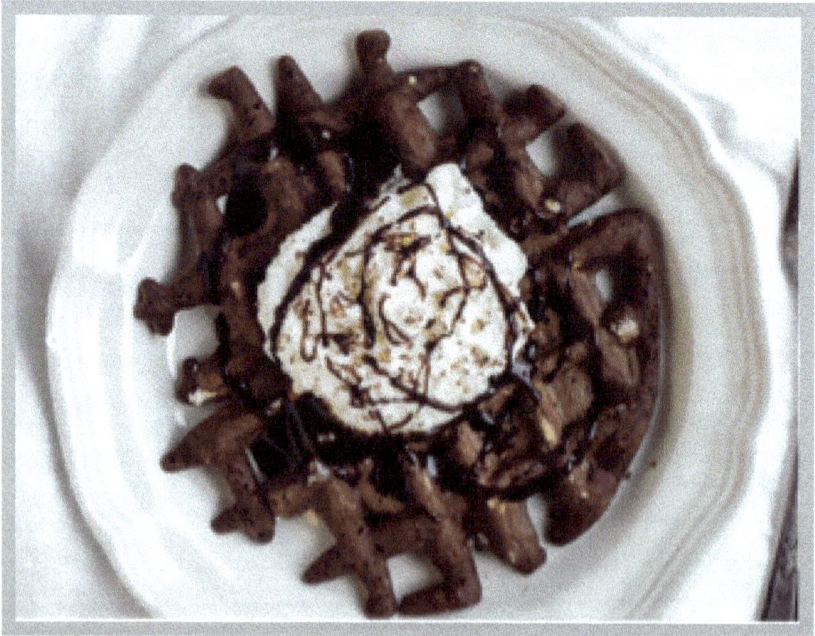

PREPARATION TIME: 1 minute
Cooking time: 5 minutes

Ready in: 6 minutes

I<small>NGREDIENTS</small>:

1. 1 egg
    2. 1 oz cream cheese
    3. 2 tablespoons almond flour
    4. 1 tablespoon unsweetened cocoa powder
    5. 2 teaspoons monk fruit
    6. 1 teaspoon vanilla extract

I<small>NSTRUCTIONS</small>:

1. At first, preheat waffle maker to medium-high heat.

2. Then whisk together egg, cream cheese, almond flour, cocoa powder, monk fruit, and vanilla.
    3. Now pour the chaffless mixture into the center of the waffle iron.

4. Then close the waffle maker and let cook for 3-5 minutes or until waffle is golden brown and set.
    5. Final stage: remove the chaff from the waffle maker and serve.

28. KETO CHOCOLATE COOKIES

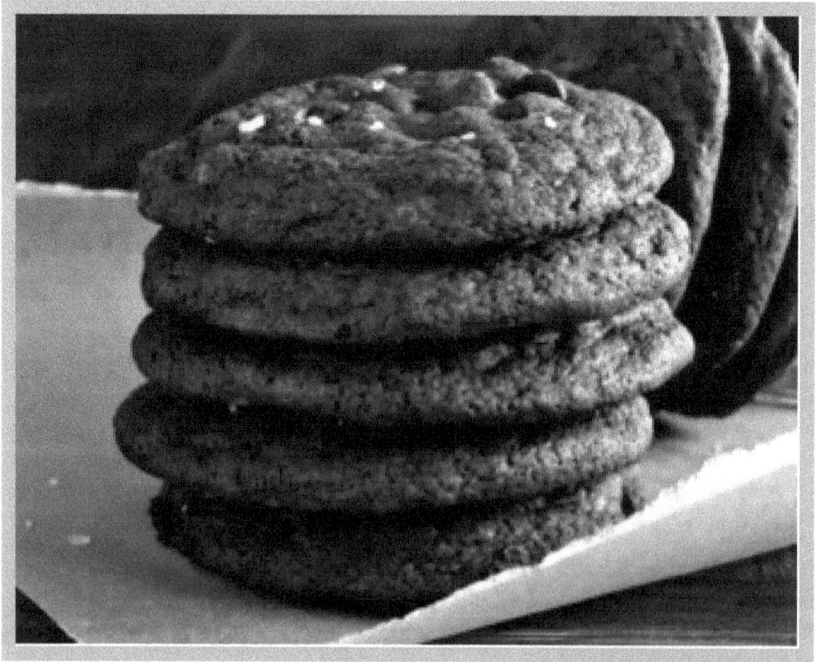

PREPARATION TIME: 15 minute

Cooking time: 10 minutes
Ready in: 25 minutes

INGREDIENTS:
1. 1 1/2 cups almond flour
2. 1/2 cup cocoa powder (unsweetened)
3. 1 teaspoon salt
4. 1 teaspoon baking soda
5. 1 1/2 sticks/12 tablespoons unsalted butter (at room temperature)
6. 3/4 cup sugar-free sweetener
7. 2 eggs
8. 1 teaspoon vanilla extract
9. 1 cup sugar-free chocolate chips
10. Garnish: Sea salt

Instructions:

1. At first, gather the ingredients and preheat the oven to 350 F and line two sheet pans with parchment paper.
2. Then add the almond flour, cocoa powder, salt, and baking soda to a bowl. Now whisk until thoroughly combined and set aside.
3. Now cream the unsalted butter and sweetener using a hand or stand mixer. Do beat until lightened in color and fluffy.
4. Do mix in the eggs and the vanilla extract.
5. Then stir in the flour mixture, just until incorporated, and then fold in the chocolate chips.
6. Now scoop out approximately 1 1/2-ounce balls onto two prepared sheet pans.
7. Then very slightly flatten the top of each cookie and sprinkle with a bit of sea salt.
8. Final stage: do bake for 8 to 10 minutes until just set and the cookies will be very soft but will firm up slightly as they cool.

29. KETO CHOCOLATE CHAFFLE RECIPE

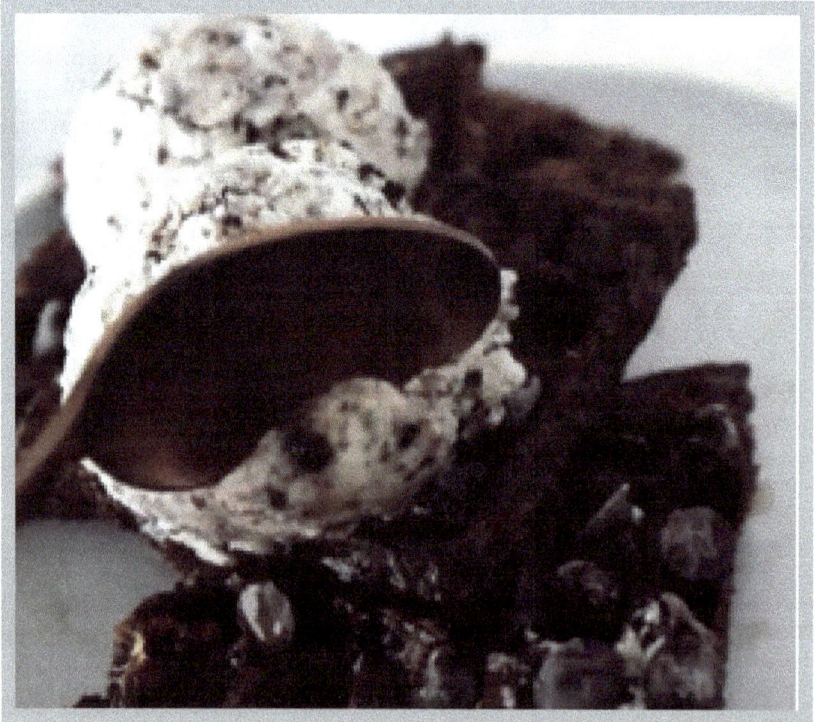

PREPARATION TIME: 5 minute
Cooking time: 5 minutes
Ready in: 10 minutes

INGREDIENTS:

1. 1 tablespoon heavy whipping cream
2. ½ teaspoon coconut flour
3. ¼ teaspoon baking powder
4. 1 large egg
5. 1 tablespoon unsweetened cocoa powder
6. Pinch of stevia extract powder

INSTRUCTIONS:

1. At first, preheat your waffle maker.

2. Take a bowl, add the egg, cocoa powder, stevia, coconut flour, baking powder, heavy whipping cream whisk it together.

3. Then pour the batter in the waffle maker and cook until ready (the time varies depending on your waffle maker).
    4. Final stage: let it cool off for about 3 minutes, it will get firmer.

30. KETO CHOCOLATE FROSTY DESSERT

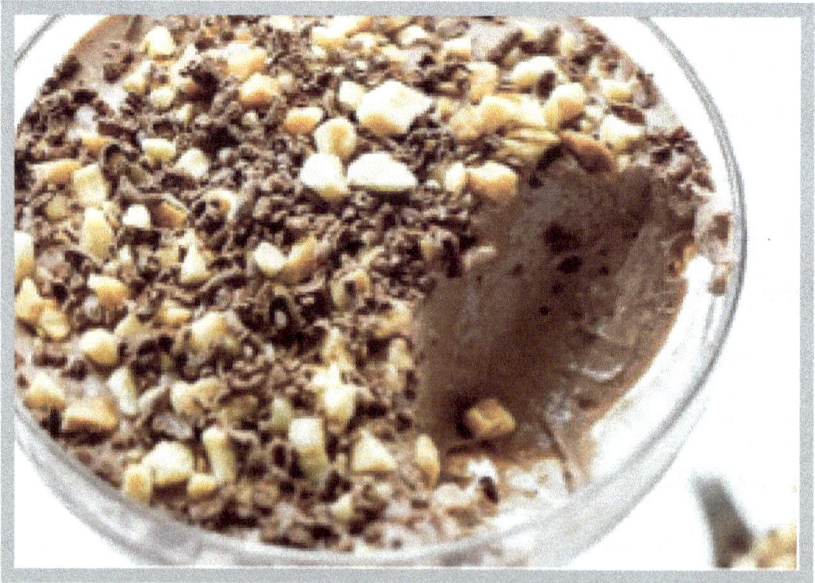

PREPARATION TIME: 4 minute
Cooking time: 6 minutes
Ready in: 10 minutes

. . .

INGREDIENTS:

1.1 CUP heavy whipping cream
2. 1 tablespoon peanut butter (or almond butter)
3. 1 teaspoon vanilla extract
4. 5 drops liquid stevia (or sweetener of your choice)
5. 2 tablespoons unsweetened cocoa powder
6. Crushed peanuts and dark chocolate shavings, for garnish

INSTRUCTIONS:

1. Take a medium bowl; use a hand mixer to beat the heavy cream for a few minutes.

2. Then add peanut butter, sweetener, and vanilla extract and blend again until the mixture becomes the consistency of thick frosting.

3. Do fold in cocoa powder and beat again until smooth, well combined and thick. Then Scoop into serving glasses and sprinkle with crushed peanuts (or almonds) and dark chocolate shavings.

4. Final stage: refrigerate until set and ready to serve – about 30 minutes. Enjoy!

www.ingramcontent.com/pod-product-compliance
Lightning Source LLC
Chambersburg PA
CBHW051039030426

42336CB00015B/2946